Intermittent Fasting For Beginners

The Essential 5:2 and 16:8 Weight Loss
Guide incl. 28 Days Weight Loss Challenge

Marc J. Williams

ISBN- 9798688700152

Table of Contents

What Is Intermittent Fasting, and How Does It Work?

Congratulations! You've decided to embark on a weight loss journey that is sure to help you feel more confident and look your best, through intermittent fasting. It is currently one of the most popular health and fitness diets in the world, and for good reason - it's great for losing weight, improving your overall health, and simplifying your lifestyle.

You've taken the first step toward changing your life for the better, and if your future self could talk to you, they'd thank you for it. However, while you may have seen and heard plenty about intermittent fasting online, it's quite likely that you aren't entirely sure about what it is. That's where this book comes in.

This chapter is all about the ins and outs of intermittent fasting. We'll cover what it is, exactly, and also how it works to keep you healthy and helps you achieve your weight loss goals. Along the way, we'll also showcase some recipes that work well with the different intermittent fasting methods.

Without further ado, let's get into the nitty-gritty.

Intermittent Fasting, or IF: What Is It?

Intermittent fasting can better be described as a pattern of eating rather than a diet. It is a method of scheduling your meals so that you're getting all you can from them, in terms of nutrients and fulfillment. The great thing about intermittent fasting is that it doesn't involve changing *what* you eat, but rather *when* you eat.

You might be wondering, "What difference does changing my eating schedule make if I'm still eating the same foods?" Plenty! One of the main appeals to intermittent fasting is that it helps you get as lean as you want without needing to go on some silly 'miracle diet' or reduce your daily caloric intake to malnourishment-inducing levels.

Most of the time, you'll actually be putting in effort to keep your caloric intake about the same as when you started the diet. Most people choose to eat larger meals in a shorter period, but we'll get into that eventually. Intermittent fasting is also a great way to maintain your muscle mass while also being able to reduce your weight.

Perhaps the most significant appeal to intermittent fasting is its extreme simplicity: it's one of the simplest plans out there for reducing your weight while also maintaining any muscles you might have since it involves very little change in behavior. This means it fits nicely into the category of 'simple enough to be doable, while impactful enough to be worth doing.'

The practice of fasting has been around throughout all the evolutionary stages of man. Prehistoric hunters and gatherers weren't able to take a walk to their local supermarkets back in their day, nor did they have refrigerators, let alone enough food to store away. Sometimes, they weren't able to find anything to eat at all.

In order to adapt, humans evolved to be able to survive without food for extended periods, and function normally. Nowadays, fasting is more of a religious practice, but as you'll soon see, it has some nice health benefits as well. Conventional intermittent fasting methods include fasting for 24 hours two times a week or fasting for 16 hours a day. The latter is more common.

How Does It Work?

It is important to understand the difference between the fasting state and the feeding state so that you can understand how intermittent fasting promotes weight loss. When your body is digesting food and absorbing its nutrients, it is in the fed state. This state usually begins when you start eating, and persists for about four or five hours, throughout the process of your body digesting the food and absorbing its nutrients. It is quite challenging for your body to burn fat while it's in the fed state because your levels of insulin will be high.

Once the fed state has been completed, your body will shift into a state known as the postabsorptive state - essentially the state your body is in when it is not processing a meal. This state lasts for about nine to twelve hours after a meal, which is also about the time that you enter the fasted state. Insulin levels are low in this state, which makes it much easier for your body to burn fat.

The fasted state also allows your body to burn fat that it otherwise was not able to while it was in the fed state. Since it takes about twelve hours for the body to enter the fasted state, it's quite rare that we burn fat during this time. This is one of the main reasons why you'll notice yourself start to lose weight while intermittent fasting, without really changing the things you eat, how often you exercise, or how much you eat. When you fast, you put your body in a state of fat-burning that it does not normally enter when you eat on a regular schedule.

Starting to get the intermittent fasting picture? Great!

The Benefits

Sure, losing weight is pretty great, but that's not the only benefit to intermittent fasting. Here are a few more:

You'll Live Longer

As you probably likely already know, shedding a few pounds will inevitably improve your overall health, which will subsequently extend your life expectancy. Scientists have known for decades that reducing your daily caloric intake is one of the many ways that you can extend your life. When you think about it logically, it makes sense - your body will find ways to live when you're starving.

But who wants to starve themselves just so they can live for a few more years? Most people want to *enjoy* the limited time they have on this earth, and starving doesn't sound all that enjoyable, at least not to us. One of the best parts of intermittent fasting is that it triggers many of the mechanisms within our bodies that a reduced caloric intake triggers.

Basically, you get to live longer and don't have to starve yourself for it. In 1945, scientists discovered that the lifespan of a mouse could be lengthened using intermittent fasting. Another study that was conducted more recently concluded that alternate-day intermittent fasting also resulted in increased life expectancies.

You'll Enjoy a Simpler Day

Many people these days are interested in changing their behaviors, reducing stress, and simplifying their daily lives. Intermittent fasting can provide these simplicities that many people crave in an enjoyable way. When you use intermittent fasting, you won't have to worry about making breakfast in the mornings, which is stressful in and of itself.

If you're someone that doesn't have a problem with cooking and enjoys eating, then the whole 'three meals a day' routine probably isn't a problem for you. But, intermittent fasting will allow you to eat one less meal each day, which means there's one less meal to plan a day, one less meal to cook, and one less meal to stress about. Life becomes simpler, and thus, less stressful.

Intermittent Fasting Is Far Easier than Any Diet

One of the biggest reasons that all the other diets you've tried have failed is not because you started eating the wrong foods, but because you weren't adhering to the diet long enough. It has much less to do with nutrition, and more to do with your behaviors.

That's where intermittent fasting comes in. It is extremely easy to enact once you unlearn the idea that you have to eat regularly. One study, which was conducted by the National Library of Medicine, discovered that intermittent fasting proved to be an effective method for losing weight in obese adults, and found that subjects were able to adapt to an intermittent fasting routine very quickly.

It's easier to think about starting a diet than actually starting one. Intermittent fasting is the exact opposite - it can be difficult to wrap your head around, but starting it is rather easy.

If you're reading this, then you've probably thought about starting a diet before. When you find a diet that seems to promise everything you're looking for, you often think that starting it will be a piece of cake, no pun intended. But when you start to get into it, things get rough, and you begin to miss the foods you enjoyed the most - fried chicken, tacos, spaghetti.

You'll also find yourself spending much less money on food, and you also won't be hungry as often. Even though getting over the idea of not being able to eat for a while, after you've begun intermittent fasting, you'll never look back.

Reduced Cancer Risk

To be fair, this one *is* debatable, since there has not been much research regarding the relationship between fasting and cancer, but early findings tend toward being more positive. A study done by the National Library of Medicine involving ten cancer patients suggested that fasting before a chemotherapy session can reduce the side effects of the treatment.

This claim is also backed by a different study, also conducted by the National Library of Medicine. In it, cancer patients used alternate day fasting, and it was discovered that fasting before a chemotherapy session resulted in increased cure rates and decreased deaths.

And finally, the American Journal of Clinical Nutrition analyzed many studies regarding disease and fasting and learned that fasting is not only capable of reducing the risk of cancer, but cardiovascular disease as well.

How Does Intermittent Fasting Affect Your Hormones?

There are quite a few things that happen to your body on the molecular and cellular level when you fast. For example, your body will begin to adjust its hormone levels once you've started to fast, in order to make your stored body fat more accessible. Your cells will also activate some important processes to repair and change your gene expressions.

The *Human Growth Hormone (HGH)* begins to soar, and they can increase as much as five times their usual levels. This helps promote fat loss and also muscle gain, amongst other benefits.

As we've mentioned earlier, your body's *insulin* changes as well. Your sensitivity to insulin will improve, while insulin levels will drop quite significantly, which results in more body fat becoming accessible. When you fast, your cells will begin to repair themselves, including a process including autophagy. Autophagy is the process of cells digesting and removing old, detrimental proteins that accumulate within cells.

In the next chapter, we'll take a look at some intermittent fasting methods and how they can promote weight loss.

Fasting Methods and How They Promote Weight Loss

So, we've covered the basics of intermittent fasting, how it works, and how it affects your body. Now it's time to take a look at some of the different fasting methods, how they work, and how they promote weight loss. You've probably seen some numbers and ratios thrown around, like 5:2 and 16:8, but you might not know what they really mean.

The ratios refer to the number of days or hours that are spent eating in one cycle, as well as how many days or hours are spent fasting. With the ratio of 5:2, five out of seven days a week are spent eating, while two out of seven days a week are spent fasting, etc.

Daily Intermittent Fasting

Most people choose to follow the Leangains intermittent fasting model, which involves a period of 16 hours spent fasting, followed by a period of 8 hours spent eating. Martin Berkhan was the man who popularized this fasting method, which originated on the Leangains website.

When you start your 8 hour eating period does not matter. You could start at 10 am and end at 6 pm, or begin at 6 pm and end at 2 am. It's entirely up to you. The only thing that matters is that you're fasting for 16 hours of the day, and eating for the 8 remaining hours. Of course, you won't be eating for 8 hours straight; you'll just have to eat enough to fill yourself during those 8 hours.

Since you'll be doing daily intermittent fasting every day, hence the name, getting into the routine of it becomes extremely easy. At the moment, you might be eating at the same time every day without even realizing it. Intermittent fasting is essentially the same, but you'll have to teach yourself to refrain from eating at certain times, which is much easier than it sounds.

This fasting schedule does come with one disadvantage, though. With it, you'll likely be cutting out one or two meals from your day, which can make it challenging to get enough calories in your body throughout the week. It basically becomes difficult to learn to eat larger meals regularly. The result is usually a reduction in weight, which, depending on your goals, can either be a good thing or a bad thing.

Weekly Intermittent Fasting

This fasting method is one of the best ways to get started with intermittent fasting, as you can do it once a week or once a month. Fasting occasionally has been proven to provide many of the fasting benefits that we have already discussed, so even if you aren't using fasting as a way to reduce your caloric intake, it still provides many other benefits.

For example, if you were to fast for one day a week, you could start at dinner time on a Monday, say 8 pm. You would then fast until 8 pm the next day, which would be Tuesday. You could then resume your eating schedule as normal for the rest of the week until you get to 8 pm the following Monday, where the cycle would start again.

The main advantage of this method of fasting is that you're able to eat almost every day, save for one day, while still receiving the benefits of fasting. However, you are much less likely to lose weight with this method, since you will only be cutting out two meals each week, so it's best to use this fasting method if you aren't trying to lose weight, or if you want to bulk up.

One of the greatest benefits that this method provides is that it helps you get past that mental block of 'if I don't eat for one day, I'll die.' You won't. You'll soon learn that after you've fasted once, fasting again becomes easier than ever.

Alternate Day Fasting

As the name suggests, this fasting method involves fasting for longer periods on different days during the week. For example, you could eat dinner on Monday night, around 8 pm, and then fast until 8 pm the next day, Tuesday. You would then eat all of Wednesday, and after Wednesday's dinner, you would start another 24-hour fast. The cycle repeats like this.

This will allow you to fast for extended periods more consistently, while also allowing you to at least once a day. This is the intermittent fasting method that is used most frequently for research purposes but isn't that popular amongst actual practitioners of intermittent fasting. Don't feel pressured to try it if it does not appeal to you.

The main benefit to this method of intermittent fasting is that you'll be in the fasted state, which we discussed in the previous chapter, for longer than the first method of intermittent fasting, the Leangains style. This could, in theory, boost the benefits of intermittent fasting. In practice, it's a different story.

The main concern is being able to eat enough during the days that you are eating. Most people find that teaching yourself to eat regularly is much more difficult than teaching yourself not to eat at certain times. You might be able to pig out for one meal, but when you have to start doing so every day, you have to start doing plenty of planning, cooking and eating.

This results in weight loss, since most people that give this style of intermittent fasting a shot don't change their meal sizes, but are eating fewer meals each week. If losing weight is a goal of yours, then this is generally not a problem. Even if your weight is not a concern of yours, then following one of the two fasting methods we mentioned previously shouldn't be a problem.

But, if you choose to use this method, you'll be fasting for entire days, multiple times every week. That means it's going to be pretty challenging to eat enough on the days that you can eat to make up for the days you didn't. That's why we recommend trying one of the previous methods before you attempt this one.

The Warrior Diet

The Warrior Diet is a more extreme method of intermittent fasting and was created by Ori Hofmekler in 2001. He is a former member of the Israeli Special Forces and made his transition to the nutrition and fitness field after his time there. As you may have guessed, the Warrior Diet is based on the eating habits of ancient warriors, who would eat very little throughout the day, and then feast at night.

Ori suggests that this diet is meant to improve the way we eat, perform, look, and feel, but stressing the body via reduced food consumption, which is supposed to trigger our survival instincts. Here's the catch: Ori acknowledges that this diet is based on his own observations and beliefs, and not on science alone.

The people that choose to follow this method of intermittent fasting undereat for 20 hours, then eat as much as they want for the other 4 hours of the day. During the fasting period, you are encouraged to eat small portions of raw vegetables and fruits, hard-boiled eggs, and dairy products, and lots of non-calorie drinks as well.

After your 20 hours of fasting, you basically have free reign to eat whatever you want, but it's recommended that you eat healthy, unprocessed, and organic foods during this feasting time. People that follow this fasting method have acclaimed that they've lost weight, burned fat, experienced better concentration, higher energy levels, and even increased cell repair.

How Does Intermittent Fasting Promote Weight Loss?

Reducing the daily caloric intake of animals has physiologically been shown to increase their life expectancies and improve their tolerance to several metabolic stressors. Even though there is plenty of evidence regarding the caloric reduction in animals, human studies, and the evidence they provide tend to be less convincing.

Many advocates for intermittent fasting believe that the stress the diet causes triggers an immune response that helps to encourage positive changes to our metabolisms, and activate cell repair. Most people have an understandable concern regarding overeating on days where you aren't fasting in order to make up the calories that were lost during the fasting period. Studies have yet to prove that this is true in comparison to other methods of losing weight.

While there have been several benefits to restricting the number of calories eaten by animals during various studies, we have yet to prove that all of the same benefits can be received by humans that practice intermittent fasting. We don't have enough research to prove whether or not intermittent fasting is better than other methods of weight loss, but we do know that it works.

Is Intermittent Fasting for You?

By now, you should be thinking about whether or not you want to start intermittent fasting. While the diet might work for some people, it isn't good for everyone. It's important to know that skipping meals at random while maintaining a diet consisting of highly processed foods will not improve your health, nor will it help you lose weight.

Even though there is no single 'correct' way to fast, a decent practice will involve putting some thought into the nutritional makeup of the food you eat, and you're going to have to put in the effort. Some people might find that intermittent is either too tedious or inconvenient to practice, while others will feel that the risks outweigh the benefits. Intermittent fasting might even be dangerous for some people.

You are safe to practice intermittent fasting if you often exercise, regularly monitor your caloric intake, have an incredibly supportive partner, live alone, and can afford to perform less-than-average at your job while adjusting to the eating plan.

You should be cautious practicing intermittent fasting if you are an athlete or a competitive sportsperson, have children and/or are married, or work in a field that requires constant performance.

Do not practice intermittent fasting if you have an eating disorder history, are pregnant, do not sleep well at night, suffer from chronic stress, or are new to exercising and dieting.

That last point is especially important. If you're new to exercising and dieting, intermittent fasting can look like the miracle diet we've already mentioned, but you will have to take care of any nutritional deficiencies you might have before you try fasting. You must make sure that your nutritional foundation is strong.

Starting Intermittent Fasting

Now it's time to actually start your intermittent fasting journey. But there are a few things you should know and do first. Instead of looking at intermittent fasting as just another challenging task that you owe yourself and your health, see it as a kind of self-experiment. It helps to break the process of starting down into small, doable tasks that you know you'll be able to finish.

During this time, you should be observing the changes that you are feeling, both physically and mentally. This is also the time that you should be deciding whether or not you really want to embark on an intermittent fasting journey. You haven't committed to anything just yet; you're still in the learning phase, which means there's still time to back out if you feel like it.

Things to Do before You Start

The first and perhaps most important thing to do before you start the process of intermittent fasting is to talk to your doctor. This is particularly important if you already have some underlying condition that might affect you, or if you're on any kind of prescribed medication. As soon as you feel sick, you need to stop.

Next, remember to keep things simple. Since intermittent fasting has nothing to do with religion or spirituality and everything to do with losing weight, you are not forbidden from consuming *everything* during your fasting periods. You're allowed to drink water, have some unsweetened tea, or black coffee. Just stay away from foods as much as you can.

Keep things easy for yourself. When your feeding time begins, eat meals that you usually would. Most people find that intermittent fasting is most effective when you maintain a diet of high-fat, low-carb, real, whole foods. Trying to catapult yourself into an extreme diet coupled with extreme fasting should not be your goal in the beginning. Your first goal is to finish a fast.

Fasting on weekdays is generally more convenient since they are much more structured and predictable than weekends. Of course, that might not be true for you. The best days for fasting are the ones where you find yourself thinking, 'Where did the time go?'. Also, remember that you have to be forgiving with yourself. You're bound to slip up sometimes, but you have to be patient enough with yourself to get back on track.

Day 1 - No Eating After Dinner

If you've done everything above, then you're ready to ease yourself into the intermittent fasting journey. To start, you have to stop eating after dinner. You probably don't really get hungry after you've had your meal at about 7 pm, but when you're lying on the couch, unwinding, watching TV, then you start to snack.

To stop this, try to substitute your cravings with a glass of water, or a cup of calming tea, rather than snacking on food. You could also try brushing your teeth earlier than usual. The minty taste can help fight your cravings, and you're also subconsciously telling yourself that you can't eat any more today; otherwise, you will have to brush your teeth again. It sounds silly, but it can really work.

If the cravings persist, you could hit the sack as a last resort. There's no time for being hungry when you are fast asleep, and chances are, you're tired anyway, since it's been a long day at work, and dinner really filled you up.

Day 2 - Postpone Breakfast

We don't mean avoid breakfast entirely. You'll get to it, just not right now. What's important now is realizing that you've just completed a twelve-hour fast. It was 7 pm the last time you ate, and now it's 7 am. That's 12 hours.

You've managed to balance your fasting and eating ratio to a perfect 50:50, which is a good thing.

You'll probably realize that it was a lot easier than you think. The only thing that you needed to do was not eat after dinner and then go to sleep. However, it's the next morning now, and as usual, it's rushed. You need to race out of the house to work, or you'll be late, so you decide to shove some toast in your mouth or take breakfast to the car.

Instead, why not delay breakfast. Eat it when you have enough time to chew. For now, have some coffee and a glass of water. We often mistake thirst for hunger. Delaying breakfast until you have time to eat it properly is no big deal. After you've gotten to work, you'll probably look at your calendar, check your emails, plan your day.

You don't have to shove breakfast into your mouth before all of this, or while all of this is happening. Before you know it, it will be 10 am, and you'll be able to have something to eat without all of the stress. Then, it's going to be 12 pm - lunchtime for most folks, but probably not for you, since you'll have eaten shortly before. Waiting to eat when you're hungry again is not a crime, so feel free to do so.

Build on these first two steps - no eating after dinner, and postponing breakfast. Then you'll be ready to move on to step three.

Day 3 - No Snacking

By this point, you will have already completed your first few 15-hour fasts. Last night you ate dinner at 7 pm, and then didn't eat again until your delayed breakfast, which was at 10 am. Now you're ready for the next task, which entails not eating again once you've had lunch. That means no snacking.

To help avoid snacking, try to remind yourself that dinner is only a few hours away. You're going to eat soon enough, and you know it. You just have to wait a little while longer, and perhaps keep yourself busy. If you're at work, then this usually isn't a problem. But, if you stay at home, then keeping yourself occupied is your responsibility. Go for a walk, do some chores, call a friend, or work on a hobby like music or art. Before you know it, it will be time to cook yourself a delicious meal for dinner, which should be around 7 pm.

Day 4 - Skip Breakfast Altogether

If you've been following the previous steps, then you will have fasted for 15 hours and did not snack the entire time. Now it's time to take it a step further and skip breakfast entirely by waiting another hour before you eat. This means that lunch will be your first meal of the day, around 11 am.

You will have practiced mindfulness when it comes to eating and will be able to perform your daily activities without needing to eat simultaneously. You'll also have avoided habitual eating, and will have experienced shorter bursts of hunger.

Then, eat dinner at 7 pm as usual.

Day 5 - Repeat

After all that, you will have fasted for 16-hours, which means you successfully completed the Daily Intermittent Fasting method, mentioned in Chapter Two. You are now ready to progress to other versions of intermittent fasting - be sure to try them all out to see which one suits you the best.

Tips for Complimenting the Diet

Following the intermittent fasting diet is a journey, and like any journey, you're going to run into some bumps along the way. You might feel like you've stopped seeing results, or you might see something online that tanks your confidence in both yourself and the diet.

That's where this chapter comes in. We're going to give you some of the best tips to keep in mind that will make your intermittent fasting and weight loss journey a little easier. Nothing worthwhile in life comes easy, but that doesn't mean that intermittent fasting needs to be impossible.

If you consider these tips and keep them in mind when the going gets tough, then you'll be rewarded with a much more fulfilling intermittent fasting experience. Without any more delay, here they are:

There Are Several Fasting Methods

Of course, you already know this, since we covered the various intermittent fasting methods in chapter two. So why are we mentioning it again? Well, it's essential for you to realize that not every fasting method is going to work for you. You might try the weekly fasting method and find that your weight hasn't changed at all.

The whole point of intermittent fasting is that it's customizable, to a certain extent. The various intermittent fasting methods exist so that you can find one that suits you and will help you reach your weight loss goals. It's no use trying one method of fasting, finding out that it doesn't work for you, and then giving up intermittent fasting altogether.

You're going to have to experiment with different methods to find the one that works for you. Don't let a little failure or setback discourage you. You've got this!

Pay Attention to Your Body

Your body will always tell you how it's feeling. If you're feeling super hungry during your fasting period, then there's no shame in eating earlier than you planned to. Re-evaluate how much you eat during the day - you might find that you'll need to get more protein and fat in during your feeding periods so that you feel more full and less hungry when you fast.

You'll know that intermittent fasting is working when you can sleep well, perform well when you work out, have a balanced feeling of energy throughout the day, and feel generally satisfied overall.

Intermittent Fasting Is Not for Everyone

Intermittent is generally considered a safe practice for most adults, but there are some people out there that should not be fasting for extended periods. We covered this briefly in the previous chapters, but pregnant women, and women that are breastfeeding, for example, will need to be nourishing their bodies as much as possible; therefore, they will need to eat more regularly.

People with health conditions, such as diabetes, or others that need to be on insulin, should avoid intermittent fasting. The elderly and people that get dizzy easily should not partake in any kind of fasting either. Be sure to check with your doctor to find out if you can practice intermittent fasting safely.

Start by Snacking Less at Night

Again, we've discussed this in the previous chapter, but it's important enough to rehash since it can make a huge difference. If you continue to eat after dinner, your body is going to take longer to digest, process, and absorb the foods, which means it will take longer for it to enter the fasting state.

This means that you're essentially delaying the benefits of intermittent fasting when you snack after dinner. If you stop the habitual snacking, you'll be able to receive all of the benefits of intermittent fasting to their fullest.

Watch Out for the Side Effects

Fasting and time-restrictive eating can come with a number of side effects, with one of the most common being dehydration. When you aren't eating, you probably aren't reminding yourself to drink water, which is when dehydration starts to kick in. It helps to keep a bottle of water nearby at all times throughout the day, so that every time you look at it, you're reminded to take a sip.

Fasting can also lead to constipation, so try to incorporate some fibrous foods into your diet during your eating periods, so that you can combat this and have healthy bowel movements.

Make Sure You're Getting Enough Calories In

Since you won't be getting your regular caloric intake throughout the day during your fasting periods, it's important that you make up for those lost calories when it's time to eat. This is where scheduling becomes most valuable, as if you've made your eating window too small, you might not have enough time to get all of those calories in.

You're Allowed to Drink

We don't mean alcohol. If you want to receive all of the benefits that intermittent fasting has to offer, then it's vital that you aren't eating food during your fasting windows. However, you are more than welcome to drink water, tea, and black coffee. In fact, it's encouraged, since they'll help you get through the day and give you a small boost throughout.

However, you should try not to drink too much coffee, as drinks with high caffeine contents can dehydrate you, especially when your body already does not have as much energy as it's used to. Alcohol is also totally off limits while you're fasting.

Make Sure Your Diet Is Balanced

Intermittent fasting does not mean 'no eating for 16 hours then eat whatever you want for 8 hours', contrary to popular belief. While you are limiting your window of eating, which can help you lose weight, it does not mean that you're allowed to binge on takeouts and ice cream.

If you're practicing intermittent fasting correctly, then you will need to be mindful of the food that you choose to put into your body during the hours that you have planned to eat. The quality of the food that you are eating is essential when it comes to staying healthy with this diet.

Does Your Lifestyle Allow This Diet?

If you're someone with plenty of friends that enjoy going out to eat or to the bar often, then intermittent fasting might not be the diet for you. You can't expect the people around you to adjust and adhere to your new patterns of eating and fasting, and you might even start to feel bummed out that you aren't able to enjoy the times you spend out with your friends and family that you used to.

Stay Away from Overeating

This is a common issue that many people that are new to intermittent fasting run the risk of encountering. You know that you are about to enter a fasting period, so you use your feeding period to load up on calories and eat as much food as you would on a typical day in just a few hours. This defeats the purpose of the intermittent fasting diet entirely.

Eat a Little Bit when You're Fasting

The general rule, when it comes to fasting, is avoiding eating anything for the entire duration of your fasting period. While this is possible, and removing food from your day entirely is something that is possible, some fasting methods allow you to eat as much as 24% of your regular daily caloric intake during your fasting periods, like the 5:2 diet, for instance.

Since you are likely still new to intermittent fasting, a great way to get started with fasting would be restricting your calories so that you are only eating small portions of food during the times when you are meant to be fasting. Not only is this safer than jumping straight into eating nothing for 24 hours, but it will also help your body adjust to eating less and less until you are finally able to go your entire fasting period without eating so much as a crumb.

Keep Yourself Busy

We mentioned this in Chapter Three. It can be pretty difficult to completely avoid eating on your fasting days, especially when the combination of hunger and boredom kicks in. It helps to go for walks, or meditate, or even take a nap, since you'll be passing the time, and hopefully, while you're doing those activities, you won't be thinking about eating.

Try not to do activities that use too much energy, like running, cycling, or swimming. Instead, opt for activities that are more mentally stimulating, like painting, playing an instrument, reading, walking, or meditating.

If You Start to Feel Sick, Stop Fasting

It is completely normal to feel hungry, tired, and even a little bit irritable when you are fasting, especially during your first few fasts when you just start intermittent fasting. What is not normal, however, if feeling unwell. You should not be feeling any kind of sick when you are fasting, and if you are, you should stop immediately.

If you want to keep yourself safe, particularly when you are just starting intermittent fasting, you should limit your fasting periods to a maximum of 24 hours - no more. You could also keep a snack nearby if you start to feel ill or faint so that you can give your body some energy to keep it going.

There are a few telling signs that you need to stop your fast and get help from a doctor or medical professional. These include things like tiredness or a sense of weakness that makes you unable to perform regular daily tasks. Unexpected feelings of discomfort and sickness are also signs that your body is taking a toll from fasting.

Eat Protein and Whole Foods

If you're reading this book, then you are most likely looking to use intermittent fasting as a way to lose weight. While that is the main purpose of the diet, it can also make you lose muscle mass as well, in addition to your body fat. One of the best ways to reduce this loss is to make sure that you are eating enough protein during your feeding periods.

Also, if you choose to eat small portions of foods during your fasting times, then you could always include some protein to help slow the muscle loss.

Protein will also help you feel more full, so you won't have to snack as much. Studies have suggested that having 30% of your calories from meals come from protein is a great way to minimize your appetite.

Don't Do Intense Workouts

You should try to make sure that the exercises you're doing while intermittent fasting are mild, and not intense. Even though some people can maintain a regular exercise routine when they are practicing intermittent fasting, that does not mean you have to, especially if you are new to fasting in general.

If you must exercise, try to ensure that you're keeping your workouts to a low intensity. Doing so will help you gauge how far you can go without harming yourself or causing any adverse side effects. Good low-intensity exercises to include are things like stretching, mild yoga, and even housework. Listen to your body - you'll know if you're struggling to exercise when intermittent fasting.

Common Concerns

After reading all of the previous chapters in this book, you might find yourself facing some concerns regarding the logistics of this diet. That's totally normal. Intermittent fasting looks quite extreme from the outside, but chances are, you've probably already fasted every now and then without even realizing it.

In this chapter, we are going to discuss some of the most frequent concerns that arise when people first start intermittent fasting. Hopefully, yours is here, and your mind will be put to rest after reading what we have to say about it. If you have a problem that we don't discuss in this chapter, then there are plenty of resources online that can help you. You could also talk to your doctor!

You Can't Give Up Breakfast. What Should You Do?

The simple answer is: eat breakfast! There's pretty much no intermittent fasting method out there that dictates which meals you must eat and which ones you must not eat. Intermittent fasting is all about the schedule one which you're eating, not which meals you're eating.

Of course, certain schedules will mean missing out on certain meals, but those skipped meals are for you to decide. If you choose to use the daily 16:8 intermittent fasting method, but you really love breakfast foods, then you could choose to fast from 7 pm until 11 am the next morning, then eat your breakfast at 11 am.

The phrase 'breakfast is the most important meal of the day' was coined by the creators of Kellogg's Corn Flakes, James Jackson, and John Kellogg as a way to get people to buy their new cereal. There's no science to support the claim, and it's not as important as you think.

"Aren't You Supposed to Eat Every Three Hours?"

You have probably heard someone say to you at least once that you're supposed to eat every three hours or eat six meals a day, or something along those lines. This was quite a popular idea for a brief time, and here's why:

When your body processes the food you eat, it burns calories. So the idea behind eating more meals in a day was that if you were eating more often, your body would be burning more calories during the day. Basically, eating more was meant to help you lose weight.

The only problem is that the number of calories that your body burns depends on the size of the meal that your body has to digest, process, and absorb. Digesting six small meals that add up to a total of 2 000 calories would use the same amount of energy as digesting two large meals consisting of 1 000 calories each.

Regardless of whether you're getting your calories from one meal or ten, you'll still be burning the same number of calories.

You Can't Imagine Going 24 Hours Without Eating

The mental barrier in your mind is the greatest challenge that you have to overcome when following an intermittent fasting diet. It sounds daunting, but when you actually start doing it, you'll quickly learn that it's nowhere near as difficult as it seems.

Fasting has been a practice in religion for centuries. Medical professionals have also endorsed the benefits that can come from fasting, way before intermittent fasting was even thought of. To put it plainly, fasting isn't a trend. It's been around forever, and it will probably be around for the foreseeable future.

Fasting also seems quite alien to most of us because many people aren't exposed to it very often. This is because food manufacturers won't be making much money if you're being told that not eating their products will make you healthier. Fasting is not something that can be marketed, and thus, you haven't been exposed to it. It only seems strange because you aren't hearing about it all the time.

Even if you don't plan on practicing intermittent fasting regularly, you should attempt to do a 24-hour fast. It's a great way to learn that you can live without food for one day. Plus, there are plenty of health benefits that can come from fasting, and once you have done it once, you'll realize that you can do it over and over again with ease.

You Ate Breakfast, Skipped Lunch, and Ate Dinner

There are two sides to this concern. On the one side, it can be beneficial, but on the other, you'll run into an issue. We'll discuss both, starting with the benefit.

If you plan to use intermittent fasting as a method for losing weight, then it should be useful to skip lunch since you will be reducing the number of calories you eat in the day. This is true even if you eat a large meal for both breakfast and dinner, since getting in the same amount of calories that you would if you ate three regular meals is difficult.

The result of skipping lunch should be that you've reduced the total number of calories eaten, which leads to some weight loss. But, one of intermittent fasting's main appeals, which we've discussed in the previous chapters, is that your body enters a fat-burning state when you fast, and during this time, you will probably burn more fat rather than lose muscle.

The problem with skipping lunch presents itself here. After you have eaten a meal, your body will take some time to digest and process the food. After that, it will enter the postabsorptive state, which was discussed in the previous chapters. This state persists for up to 12 hours, after which you will enter the fasted state.

This means that you will need to spend at least 8-12 hours without eating before you enter the fat-burning fasted state. This is the principle that intermittent fasting is based on, and is the reason that you want to fit all of your daily meals into a smaller time frame.

Even though skipping lunch would result in an overall decrease in the number of calories that you consume, which can end up helping you lose weight, you would also be spreading your meals out. This makes it difficult to enter the postabsorptive state and get to the fasted state. To receive all of intermittent fasting's benefits, you will need to fast for a minimum of 12 hours.

Recipes

Breakfast

Green Smoothie

Carbs: 6 grams
Protein: 4.2 grams
Fat: 48.2 grams
Calories: 468kcal

INGREDIENTS:

- 1 cup coconut milk
- 1 avocado
- 1 cup kale, spinach, or chard
- 1 handful of blueberries
- 1 tbsp chia seeds

INSTRUCTIONS:

1. Place all of the above ingredients into a blender, and blend until smooth. Pour into your favorite cup and enjoy!

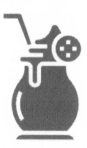

Spinach Parmesan Baked Eggs

Carbs: 5.22 grams
Protein: 13.67 grams
Fat: 15.54 grams
Calories: 215kcal

INGREDIENTS:

- 2 minced garlic cloves
- 2 teaspoons of olive oil
- ½ cups of grated parmesan cheese, fat free
- 4 cups of baby spinach
- 1 small diced tomato
- 4 eggs

INSTRUCTIONS:

1. Start by preheating your oven to 350°F / 180°C and spraying an 8 x 8 inch / 20 x 20 cm dish with nonstick spray.
2. Heat the olive oil over a medium heat in a large skillet.
3. Add the garlic and spinach when it's hot, and saute until the spinach wilts.
4. Take off the heat and drain the liquids.
5. Incorporate parmesan cheese and place the mixture on the dish evenly.
6. Create four small depressions in the spinach to place the eggs in. Crack an egg in each, and bake for 20 minutes.
7. Remove from the oven and serve with tomato.

Hummus Breakfast Bowl

Carbs: 34 grams
Protein: 14 grams
Fat: 2 grams
Calories: 354kcal

INGREDIENTS:

- 1 cup of roughly chopped kale leaves
- 2 tbsp minced bell pepper
- 1 tbsp olive oil
- ¼ cup diced roma tomato
- ¼ cup quinoa or brown rice
- 2 egg whites
- 1 tbsp hummus
- 1 tbsp sunflower seeds

INSTRUCTIONS:

1. In a large skillet, heat olive oil over medium heat.
2. Add the kale when it's hot, and saute for 4 minutes.
3. Add the peppers and tomatoes, and cook for 4 more minutes.
4. Beat the egg whites lightly and add the peppers and kale slowly, then scramble.
5. Place the quinoa or rice into a serving bowl, top with egg and vegetables.
6. Place the hummus on top and add sunflower seeds.

Mango Smoothie

Carbs: 35 grams
Protein: 12 grams
Fat: 18 grams
Calories: 340kcal

INGREDIENTS:

- ♦ 1 cup almond milk
- ♦ 2 tsp matcha
- ♦ 1 sliced mango
- ♦ 1 frozen banana
- ♦ Some ide

INSTRUCTIONS:

1. Blend all ingredients together in a blender until smooth. Serve and enjoy.

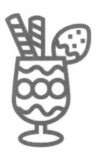

French Toast

Carbs: 42 grams
Protein: 5 grams
Fat: 16 grams
Calories: 320kcal

INGREDIENTS:

- 1 egg
- ¼ almond milk
- 1 tsp cardamom
- 1 tsp cinnamon
- 2 slices of whole wheat bread
- 1 tbsp maple syrup
- Fruit of your choice

INSTRUCTIONS:

1. Beat the eggs and almond milk together in a large bowl.
2. Add spices and continue mixing.
3. Dip your bread into the mixture and coat both sides.
4. Let the bread rest for a few minutes, then cook for 3 minutes a side in a pan.
5. Remove when golden brown, top with fruit and maple syrup, and enjoy.

Lunch

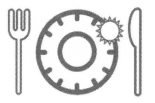

Burgers, Grass-Fed Style

Carbs: N/A
Protein: 36 grams
Fat: 30 grams
Calories: 390kcal

INGREDIENTS:

- 0.5 pound / 0.25 kg grass-fed beef
- 0.5 pound / 0.25 kg grass-fed beef liver
- ½ tsp cumin
- ½ tsp garlic powder
- Cooking oil to preference
- Salt and pepper to taste

INSTRUCTIONS:

1. Combine all ingredients in a large bowl.
2. Mold into patties of your desired size.
3. Heat cooking oil over medium-high heat in a skillet.
4. Cook the patties until preferred color and texture.

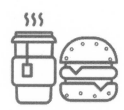

Salmon and Vegetables

Carbs: 3.3 grams
Protein: 30.6 grams
Fat: 54.7 grams
Calories: 632kcal

INGREDIENTS:

- 1 pound / 500g salmon
- 2 tbsp ghee
- 2 tbsp lemon juice, fresh
- 4 finely diced garlic cloves
- Vegetables of your choice

INSTRUCTIONS:

1. Preheat your oven to 400°F / 200°C.
2. Combine ghee, lemon juice, and garlic in a bowl. Place salmon in foil and pour the combined mixture over.
3. Wrap the salmon in the foil and place on a baking sheet.
4. Bake until salmon is fully cooked.
5. Roast vegetables alongside if you have enough space in your oven.

Fish Tacos

Carbs: 8.5 grams
Protein: 26.8 grams
Fat: 31.7 grams
Calories: 446kcal

INGREDIENTS:

- 5 fish fillets cut into strips of 2 inches / 5 cm wide
- 2 egg whites
- ¼ cup of whole wheat flour
- ¼ cup of whole wheat bread crumbs
- ¼ cup of cornmeal
- 2 tbsp of taco seasoning
- 2 tbsp of lime juice, freshly squeezed
- 8 tortillas, 8 inch / 20 cm, whole wheat or corn
- 1 cup salsa or 1 diced tomato
- 1 cup shredded cabbage or lettuce
- 1 cup Greek yogurt, non-fat

INSTRUCTIONS:

1. Preheat the oven to 450°F / 230°C.
2. Line a baking sheet with foil, and put a cooling rack on top.
3. Spray with canola or olive oil cooking spray.
4. Combine cornmeal, breadcrumbs, and taco seasoning in a small bowl.
5. Whisk lime juice and egg whites in another bowl till frothing.
6. Place flour in a third bowl.
7. Gently dip fish in until both sides are coated.
8. Dip into the egg white mixture, letting excess run off.
9. Dip both sides of fish into breadcrumbs and cornmeal mixture.
10. Place the strips on to the rack and bake until golden brown, and fish can be flaked with a fork.
11. Warm the tortillas using preferred method, keeping them warm until ready to eat.
12. Place two strips in each shell, top with lettuce / cabbage, salsa / tomato, and greek yogurt.

Turkey Burrito Skillet

Carbs: 31 grams
Protein: 30 grama
Fat: 15 grams
Calories: 379kcal

INGREDIENTS:

- 1 pound / 0.5kg ground turkey
- 1 tbsp chili powder
- 1 tbsp lime juice
- 1 tbsp ground cumin
- ¼ tsp ground black pepper
- ½ tsp kosher salt
- ¼ cup water
- 1 can black beans, drained and rinsed
- 1 cup chunky salsa, no sugar
- 4 tortillas, cut into 1 inch / 2.5cm strips
- ½ cup plain greek yogurt
- 1 cup cheddar, low fat
- ¼ fresh chopped cilantro

INSTRUCTIONS:

1. Cook ground turkey through in a large skillet.
2. As it cooks, break it into small pieces.
3. Stir in cumin, chili powder, salt, lime juice, pepper, water, beans, and salsa.
4. Bring to a boil, then let simmer for 5 minutes, until thick.
5. Remove from the heat and incorporate tortillas.
6. Top with cheddar, and cover until melted.
7. Top each serving with fresh cilantro and greek yogurt, and serve.

Baked Lemon Salmon & Asparagus in a Foil Pack

Carbs: 7 grams
Protein: 32 grams
Fat: 26 grams
Calories: 386kcal

INGREDIENTS:

- ◆ 4 salmon filets
- ◆ 1 tsp kosher salt
- ◆ 1 pound / 500g asparagus, fresh, with ends chopped off
- ◆ 2 tbsp olive oil
- ◆ ½ tsp black pepper
- ◆ 1 tbsp thyme, freshly chopped
- ◆ ¼ cup lemon juice, fresh
- ◆ 2 tbsp lemon zest
- ◆ 2 tbsp parsley, freshly chopped

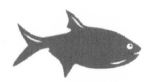

INSTRUCTIONS:

1. Preheat your oven to 400°F / 200°C.
2. Place down 4 large foil sheets on a flat surface and spray them with nonstick.
3. Evenly distribute the asparagus onto the foil side by side.
4. Use half of the salt and pepper to season.
5. Place one salmon filet on each asparagus bed.
6. Drizzle olive oil over, as well as lemon juice, then sprinkle the leftover salt and pepper, and thyme.
7. Fold the foil sheets to create a packet for the salmon, and place on a baking sheet, beside one another.
8. Bake for 15 to 20 minutes.
9. Carefully open the packets after removing from the oven.
10. Sprinkle the lemon zest over, as well as parsley, and enjoy.

Dinner

Broccoli and Chicken Stir Fry

Carbs: 15 grams
Protein: 35 grams
Fat: 18 grams
Calories: 256kcal

INGREDIENTS:

- 3 tbsp soy sauce, light
- 2 tsp sesame seeds
- 1 tbsp honey
- 2 tbsp sesame oil
- 2 tsp lemon
- 1 tbsp extra-virgin olive oil
- 1 tbsp flour or cornstarch
- 1.5 pounds / 600g cubed chicken breasts
- 1 peeled and chopped, small ginger root
- 1 coarsely chopped onion
- ¼ tsp black pepper
- 2 cups broccoli

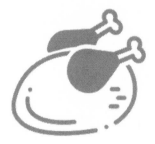

1. Whisk the honey, soy sauce, sesame oil, lemon juice, and flour together.
2. Set aside the mixture.
3. Toast the sesame seeds for two minutes in a large skillet over medium-low heat, until fragrant.
4. Place into a bowl.
5. To the same skillet, add olive oil and turn up heat to medium.
6. Cook the chicken until lightly golden.
7. Add ginger, onions, pepper, and broccoli, and saute for 5 minutes.
8. Lower the heat, add soy sauce mixture, and mix.
9. Cook until the sauce is thick, but not for longer than 5 minutes.
10. Sprinkle with sesame seeds, and serve.

Garlic & Honey Shrimp Fry

Carbs: 41 grams
Protein: 28 grams
Fat: 5 grams
Calories: 316kcal

INGREDIENTS:

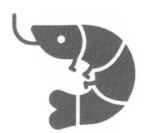

- ♦ 1 pound / 500g peeled, deveined, raw shrimp
- ♦ 1 tbsp coconut oil
- ♦ 2 minced garlic cloves
- ♦ 1 small onion, in strips
- ♦ 1 tbsp fresh minced ginger
- ♦ 1 cup peas
- ♦ 1 small red bell pepper, in strips
- ♦ 2 tbsp honey
- ♦ ½ tsp kosher salt
- ♦ 1 tbsp orange zest
- ♦ 1 tbsp soy sauce
- ♦ 2 cups cooked brown rice

INSTRUCTIONS:

1. Heat up the coconut oil in a large skillet over high heat.
2. Add shrimp when hot, half of the ginger, and half of the garlic.
3. Stir continuously, until the shrimp become firm.
4. Take the shrimp out and set aside.
5. Add bell pepper, onion, peas, and leftover ginger and garlic to the same pan.
6. Stir continuously until vegetables become soft.
7. Place the shrimp back in, season with salt and add soy sauce, honey, and orange zest.
8. Cook until everything is coated, and serve over brown rice.

Cod and Moroccan Couscous

Carbs: 31 grams
Protein: 26 grams
Fat: 5 grams
Calories: 279kcal

INGREDIENTS:

- 1 can of diced tomatoes
- ½ cup of low sodium, fat free chicken broth
- Chopped green chilies to taste
- ¾ cup Moroccan couscous
- 1 tbsp + 2 tsp olive oil
- Sea salt and black pepper to taste
- 1 tbsp lemon juice, freshly squeezed
- 4 cod fillets

INSTRUCTIONS:

1. Add 2 teaspoons of olive oil, the chicken broth, and the diced tomatoes with the juice to a medium pot.
2. Place on medium-high heat and boil.
3. Add salt, pepper, and couscous.
4. Stir, cover, and remove from heat.
5. Let couscous sit while preparing cod.
6. Use salt and pepper to season cod, then add the leftover oil to a nonstick skillet.
7. Place on medium-high heat and cook until fillets can be broken apart with a fork. Should take about 3 minutes on each side.
8. Serve with couscous and enjoy!

Chicken Parm Stuffed Peppers

Carbs: 23.3 grams
Protein: 37.9 grams
Fat: 25.9 grams
Calories: 457kcal

INGREDIENTS:

- ½ cup freshly grated parmesan
- 3 cup shredded mozzarella
- 1 ½ cup marinara
- 3 minced garlic cloves
- Kosher salt
- Crushed red pepper flakes
- Some black pepper
- 4 bell peppers, cut in half and insides removed
- 12 oz. / 350g diced chicken, cooked all the way through

INSTRUCTIONS:

1. Preheat oven to 400°F / 200°C.
2. Combine mozzarella, garlic, parmesan, marinara, red pepper flakes, and parsley in a bowl, and season with salt and pepper.
3. Combine, and add cooked chicken, coating fully.
4. Place the mixture into the bell peppers and use the rest of the mozzarella to top.
5. Bake until the peppers are tender, usually for about an hour. Serve and enjoy.

Zucchini Enchiladas

Carbs: 21 grams
Protein: 15 grams
Fat: 18.7 grams
Calories: 346kcal

INGREDIENTS:

- 1 chopped large onion
- 1 tbsp olive oil
- 2 tsp cumin
- 2 minced garlic cloves
- 2 tsp chili powder
- 3 cup shredded rotisserie chicken
- Kosher salt
- 4 large, split zucchini
- 1 ⅓ cup red enchilada sauce
- 1 cup shredded cheddar
- 1 cup shredded monterey jack
- Fresh cilantro
- Sour cream

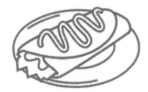

1. Preheat oven to 350°F / 180°C.
2. Heat oil over medium heat in large skillet.
3. Add and cook onion until soft.
4. Add cumin, garlic, chili powder, and salt.
5. Cook for a minute, then add 1 cup enchilada sauce and chicken.
6. Stir until cooked.
7. Peel this slices of zucchini on a cutting board, and lay three slices, overlapping them slightly.
8. Top with one spoon of the chicken mixture.
9. Roll and move to a baking dish.
10. Repeat with the rest of the mixture and zucchini.
11. Spoon the rest of the enchilada sauce over the zucchini enchiladas, and top with both cheeses.
12. Bake for 20 minutes, until enchiladas are warm inside and cheese is melted. Serve and enjoy.

28 - Day Weight Loss Challenge, Plan with Recipes

Participating in a weight loss challenge can be a great way to get started with intermittent fasting. It can help you determine whether or not the fasting method that you have chosen is working for you, and can also help you see what you need to change about your diet.

In this brief chapter, we'll take you through the full 28 days of this weight loss challenge, provide you with some tasty and nutrient-packed recipes to help you lose weight, and outline the plan you should be following. Hopefully, by the end, you'll have lost at least a little bit of weight, and will be fully confident in the power of intermittent fasting.

Let's get started!

Plan

Rule #1 - Try to follow the recipes as closely as possible. If you don't have access to all of the ingredients, no worries. There are plenty of resources online to help you find substitutes.

Rule #2 - This weight loss challenge follows the 50:50 intermittent fasting method. This means 12 hours of the day are spent eating, while the other 12 hours are spent fasting. We recommend eating from 9 am to 9 pm.

Rule #3 - Alternate light cardio with light weight training to boost the fat-burning process.

DAY 1

Breakfast - Avocado Toast

Carbs: 27 grams
Protein: 18 grams
Fat: 16 grams
Calories: 330kcal

INGREDIENTS:

- 2 slices of whole wheat bread
- 1 fresh avocado
- 2 tsp low fat cream cheese
- Sea salt and ground pepper to taste

INSTRUCTIONS:

1. Lightly toast the slices of whole wheat bread in a pan or in a toaster until desired.
2. While the bread is toasting, prepare your avocado by cutting it in half, scooping the contents out, and smoothing into a paste.
3. When the bread is fully toasted, place on a plate.
4. Spread avocado evenly on both slices, top with 1 teaspoon of cream cheese on eat, then season with salt and pepper.

Lunch - Burgers, Grass-Fed Style (See page 52)
Dinner - Broccoli and Chicken Stir Fry (See page 60)

DAY 2

Breakfast - Spinach Parmesan Baked Eggs (See page 47)
Lunch - Shrimp and Avocado Salad, with Seafood Sauce

Carbs: 4 grams
Protein: 27 grams
Fat: 33 grams
Calories: 426kcal

INGREDIENTS:

Salad:

♦ 2 small gem lettuces

♦ 1 pounds / 500g peeled, cooked shrimp

♦ 1 large avocado

♦ 1 tbsp lemon juice

♦ 1tbsp cilantro, chopped

♦ Sea salt and pepper to taste

Seafood Sauce:

♦ 2 tbsp ketchup, sugar-free

♦ ½ cup low-fat mayo

♦ 1 tsp Worcestershire sauce

♦ Cayenne pepper to taste

1. Place all sauce ingredients into a small bowl. Whisk until well combined and smooth, then pour into a serving bowl.
2. Use salt and pepper to season shrimp.
3. Slice avocado and toss in lemon juice to prevent browning.
4. Tear up lettuce and spread onto a serving bowl or tray.
5. Scatter shrimp, then place avocado around the shrimp.
6. Sprinkle with coriander, and serve with lemon wedges.

Dinner - Garlic & Honey Shrimp Fry (See page 62)

DAY 3

Breakfast - Hummus Breakfast Bowl (See page 48)
Lunch - Salmon and Vegetables (See page 53)
Dinner - Salmon BLT

Carbs: 6 grams
Protein: 44 grams
Fat: 65 grams
Calories: 789kcal

INGREDIENTS:

- 1 small salmon fillet
- 1 whole wheat burger bun
- 1 tbsp avocado oil
- 2 leaves lettuce
- 2 slices bacon
- 1 red onion, sliced
- 1 tomato slice
- 1 tbsp mayo

INSTRUCTIONS:

1. Place a skillet over a high heat.
2. Use salt and pepper to season salmon.
3. Add oil to the skillet and cook bacon until desired.
4. Sear the salmon for 5 minutes until golden brown.
5. Flip the skin side up and cook for another 2 minutes.
6. Remove and set aside. Slice the bun in half and place ingredients in the desired order. Enjoy!

DAY 4

Breakfast - Italian Melt Omelet

Carbs: 4 grams
Protein: 37 grams
Fat: 43 grams
Calories: 555kcal

INGREDIENTS:

- 6 cherry tomatoes
- 1 tbsp + 1 tsp olive oil
- 2 slices prosciutto di Parma
- 1 tbsp basil, freshly chopped
- Some fresh mozzarella slices
- 3 large eggs
- Salt and pepper to taste

INSTRUCTIONS:

1. Pour the tablespoon of oil into a pan and heat over medium heat.
2. Cut tomatoes into quarters while the oil heats, chop the prosciutto and mozzarella into small pieces, and cut the tomatoes.
3. Break the eggs into a bowl, season, and beat until frothy.
4. Pour into the pan, let cook, then gently lift with a spatula.
5. Cook until almost all the way set, then add prosciutto, mozzarella, basil, and tomatoes on one side of the omelet.
6. Fold the omelet over, remove from the heat, and let sit. Drizzle leftover oil over. Serve and enjoy!

Lunch - Fish Tacos (See page 54)
Dinner - Cod and Moroccan Couscous (See page 64)

DAY 5

Breakfast - Mango Smoothie (See page 49)
Lunch - Chicken Salad

Carbs: 3.3 grams
Protein: 35 grams
Fat: 44 grams
Calories: 553kcal

INGREDIENTS:

- 3 slices of bacon
- 2 chicken breasts, boneless
- 4 cups leafy greens of your choice
- 1 sliced avocado
- 4 tbsp ranch dressing
- Salt and pepper

INSTRUCTIONS:

1. Preheat your oven to 400°F / 200°C.
2. Season the chicken breasts on all sides with salt and pepper.
3. Grease a small skillet, and place the chicken on the pan when it's hot.
4. Cook on high until crispy.
5. Flip the chicken and repeat.
6. Transfer to the oven. Bake for 15 minutes.
7. Then, bake bacon for 10 minutes until golden brown and crispy.
8. Transfer chicken to cutting board when finished and let sit for 5 minutes.
9. Slice the avo and chicken, and put the salad together. Serve and enjoy.

Dinner - Chicken Parm Stuffed Peppers (See page 66)

DAY 6

Breakfast - French Toast (See page 50)
Lunch - Turkey Burrito Skillet (See page 56)
Dinner - Steak Taco Bowl

Carbs: 9 grams
Protein: 34 grams
Fat: 56 grams
Calories: 702kcal

INGREDIENTS:

- 1 small steak of your choice
- 1 cup cauliflower rice
- 1 tbsp butter
- 1 tsp lime juice
- 2 tbsp minced cilantro
- Salt and pepper
- 1 tbsp sour cream
- ½ sliced avocado
- ½ sliced jalapeno
- ¼ cup tomato salsa
- 2 thinly sliced radishes

INSTRUCTIONS:

1. Melt butter over medium-high heat in a skillet.
2. Use salt and pepper to season steak, and sear for 8 minutes a side.
3. Place on cutting board to rest.
4. Mix lime juice, cilantro, and cooked cauliflower rice in a bowl.
5. Top with remaining ingredients, then add thin steak slices on top.

DAY 7

Breakfast - Breakfast Burrito
Carbs: 6.4 grams
Protein: 23 grams
Fat: 52 grams
Calories: 614kcal

INGREDIENTS:

- ½ cup tomato salsa
- 2 tortillas
- 1 tbsp almond milk, unsweetened
- 3 large eggs
- 1 tbsp butter
- Salt and pepper
- ½ cup shredded cheddar
- 3 tbsp sour cream
- ½ sliced avocado

INSTRUCTIONS:

1. Warm up tortillas in a pan until soft.
2. Whisk almond milk and eggs into a bowl until scrambled.
3. Add salt and pepper.
4. Add oil to frying pan over medium heat.
5. Add eggs and cook.
6. Stir gently until barely cooked.
7. Lay down tortillas, place cheese, eggs, avo, sour cream, and salsa.
8. Roll up and enjoy.

Lunch - Baked Lemon Salmon & Asparagus in a Foil Pack (See page 57)

Dinner - Zucchini Enchiladas (See page 67)

DAY 8

Breakfast - Avocado Toast (See page 71)
Lunch - Tricolore Salad

Carbs: 9 grams
Protein: 19 grams
Fat: 51 grams
Calories: 581kcal

INGREDIENTS:

- ◆ 1 large avo
- ◆ 4 medium tomatoes
- ◆ 4.4 oz. / 125g soft salad mozzarella

- ◆ 6 olives
- ◆ 2 tbsp olive oil
- ◆ 2 tbsp pesto
- ◆ Salt and pepper

INSTRUCTIONS:

1. Wash tomatoes, then slice.
2. Slice avocado, halve olives, and add everything to a bowl.
3. Add mozzarella, olive oil, and pesto.
4. Season with salt and pepper to taste, serve, and enjoy.

Dinner - Salmon BLT (See page 74)

DAY 9

Breakfast - Green Smoothie (See page 46)
Lunch - Shrimp and Avocado Salad, with
Seafood Sauce (See page 72)
Dinner - Mexican Tacos

Carbs: 7 grams
Protein: 28 grams
Fat: 54 grams
Calories: 658kcal

INGREDIENTS:

- ◆ 4 taco shells
- ◆ 1 pound / 500g ground beef
- ◆ 2 garlic cloves
- ◆ 1 finely diced white onion
- ◆ ½ tsp cumin
- ◆ 1 tsp chili powder
- ◆ 2 tbsp ghee
- ◆ 1 tbsp tomato puree, unsweetened
- ◆ 1 cup water
- ◆ Sea salt and black pepper
- ◆ 1 diced avocado
- ◆ 1 small lettuce head
- ◆ 1 cup cherry tomatoes

INSTRUCTIONS:

1. Place chopped onion in a greased pan and fry over medium-high heat.
2. When brown, add beef and cook until redness disappears.
3. Add cumin and chili powder, mix, then add water and tomato puree.
4. Add salt and pepper and mix thoroughly.
5. When fully cooked, set aside and prepare taco shells.
6. Wash all vegetables, chop the tomatoes, avocado, and lettuce as desired.
7. Place the meat down first, then the tomatoes, lettuce, avocado, and other optional toppings.

DAY 10

Breakfast - Vanilla Smoothie

Carbs: 7 grams

Protein: 35 grams

Fat: 45 grams

Calories: 577kcal

INGREDIENTS:

- ½ coconut milk or soured cream
- 2 large eggs
- 1 tbsp extra virgin coconut oil
- ¼ cup whey, plain or vanilla
- 5 drops of Stevia extract
- 1 tsp vanilla extract, sugar free
- ¼ cup of water
- Some ice cubes

INSTRUCTIONS:

1. Add all ingredients to a blender, blend until smooth, and enjoy!

Lunch - Salmon and Vegetables (See page 53)

Dinner - Cod and Moroccan Couscous (See page 64)

DAY 11

Breakfast - Spinach Parmesan Baked Eggs (See page 47)
Lunch - Sardine Stuffed Avocado

Carbs: 6 grams
Protein: 27 grams
Fat: 52 grams
Calories: 634kcal

INGREDIENTS:

- 1 drained tin of sardines
- 1 large avocado
- 1 spring onion
- 1 tbsp mayo
- ¼ tsp turmeric
- 1 tbsp lemon juice, fresh
- Salt and pepper

INSTRUCTIONS:

1. Place the sardines into a bowl and use a fork to break them apart.
2. Add the turmeric, spring onion, and mayo to the bowl.
3. Scoop out the avocado, making sure to leave some in the shell, and add it to the bowl, and mix until well combined.
4. Put the mixture into the avocado shell, and enjoy.

Dinner - Broccoli and Chicken Stir Fry (See page 60)

DAY 12

Breakfast - Hummus Breakfast Bowl (See page 48)
Lunch - Turkey Burrito Skillet (See page 56)
Dinner - Bacon, Chicken, and Spinach Salad

Carbs: 3 grams
Protein: 35 grams
Fat: 44 grams
Calories: 553kcal

INGREDIENTS:

- 5 bacon slices
- 2 chicken breasts
- 1 fresh spinach pack
- 2 tbsp olive oil
- 4 sun-dried tomato pieces
- 1 minced garlic clove
- 1 cup low-fat ranch
- 1 cup mushroom slices
- Small bunch of basil

INSTRUCTIONS:

1. Cube the chicken, and dice the garlic finely.
2. Add olive heal to a frying pan, heat it up, and brown the chicken and the garlic.
3. When done, place in a bowl, and fry the bacon.
4. Place the bacon and the chicken in a big bow, and add raw mushroom slices.
5. Add a handful of spinach and the basil, and mix.
6. Place the rest of the spinach in a bowl and lay the chicken mix on top.
7. Sprinkle tomato on top, and dress with ranch.

DAY 13

Breakfast - Bacon, Eggs, and Avocado
Carbs: 5 grams
Protein: 30 grams
Fat: 25 grams
Calories: 362kcal

INGREDIENTS:

- 2 eggs, desired size
- 1 medium avocado
- 2 slices of bacon
- 1 slice whole wheat bread
- ½ diced garlic clove
- 1 tbsp olive oil
- Salt and pepper to taste

INSTRUCTIONS:

1. Add olive oil to a frying pan, and saute garlic for 1 - 2 minutes.
2. Remove, and crack eggs into pan.
3. Fry as desired, and remove when done.
4. Fry bacon in the same oil.
5. While the bacon is cooking, place whole wheat bread into oven or toaster to toast.
6. Slice the avocado, and place on a plate.
7. Place cooked eggs and bacon onto the same plate, as well as toasted bread.
8. Season with salt and pepper, and enjoy.

Lunch - Fish Tacos (See page 54)
Dinner - Garlic & Honey Shrimp Fry (See page 62)

DAY 14

Breakfast - Mango Smoothie (See page 49)
Lunch - Bacon Wrapped Chicken Parcels

Carbs: 2 grams
Protein: 57 grams
Fat: 30 grams
Calories: 492kcal

INGREDIENTS:

- ◆ 7.1 oz. / 200g cream cheese
- ◆ 4 chicken breasts
- ◆ 2 tbsp chopped herbs
- ◆ ½ grated parmesan
- ◆ 8 thin bacon slices
- ◆ Salt and pepper to taste

INSTRUCTIONS:

1. To prep cheese stuffing, place parmesan, cream cheese, and parsley into a bowl and mix well.
2. Divide into four portions and roll into logs the size of the chicken using cling wrap.
3. Place in the freezer for about 30 minutes.
4. Preheat oven to 400°F / 200°C.
5. Line a baking tray and cut a gap into each one, not all the way through, just about half way.
6. Place the cheese mixture into each.
7. Wrap each piece of chicken in two bacon slices.
8. Bake for 30 minutes, or until everything is golden brown.
9. Garnish with parsley when serving.

Dinner - Cod & Moroccan Couscous (See page 64)

DAY 15

Breakfast - French Toast (See page 50)
Lunch - Turkey Burrito Skillet (See page 56)
Dinner - Chorizo, Chicken, and Avocado Salad

Carbs: 8 grams
Protein: 44 grams
Fat: 43 grams
Calories: 616kcal

INGREDIENTS:

- ◆ 1 tsp ghee
- ◆ 2 chicken breasts
- ◆ 1 finely diced red onion
- ◆ 2.1 oz. / 60g chorizo or pepperoni slices
- ◆ ½ avocado
- ◆ 1 cup sugar snap peas
- ◆ 1 tbsp + 1 tsp olive oil
- ◆ 3 tbsp pine nuts
- ◆ ½ tbsp red wine vinegar
- ◆ 1 tbsp capers
- ◆ 2 tbsp chopped chives and mints
- ◆ Bunch of parsley
- ◆ Salt and pepper

1. Use 1 teaspoon of olive oil to season chicken, along with salt and pepper.
2. Use olive oil to grease pan.
3. Fry chicken on medium heat for 2 minutes for each side, then for 5 minutes on each side again.
4. Remove from the pan and let cool slightly.
5. Chop chorizo and lightly fry on medium heat for 2 minutes.
6. If chorizo is raw, cook for longer.
7. Add 1 tablespoon of olive oil to a clean pan and saute onions for 4 minutes until soft.
8. Remove from heat and stir in red wine vinegar.
9. Add the chorizo and its oil.
10. Boil sugar snap peas for a minute then plunge into cold water.
11. Take out of the water and halve them.
12. Chop herbs, stir peas, onion mix, and chorizo and top with chicken, avocado, pine nuts, and black pepper.
13. Serve and enjoy!

DAY 16

Breakfast - Chocolate Coconut Smoothie

Carbs: 7 grams

Protein: 12 grams

Fat: 43 grams

Calories: 510kcal

INGREDIENTS:

- 1 ¼ cup almond milk
- ½ large avo
- 1 tbsp chia seeds
- ¼ cup coconut cream
- 1 tsp coconut oil
- 1 ½ cacao powder
- 1 tbsp almond butter

INSTRUCTIONS:

1. Place all ingredients into a blender and blend until smooth and creamy.

   Best served right away, and be sure to thin with water if too thick.

Lunch - Baked Lemon Salmon & Asparagus in a Foil Pack (See page 57)

Dinner - Chicken Parm Stuffed Peppers (See page 66)

DAY 17

Breakfast - Green Smoothie (See page 46)
Lunch - Tuna Bowl

Carbs: 6 grams
Protein: 44 grams
Fat: 71 grams
Calories: 866kcal

INGREDIENTS:

- 1 tuna steak
- Sea salt
- 1 tsp sesame seeds
- ½ avocado
- 1 tsp ghee
- 1 tbsp mayo
- 10 black olives, pitted
- 1 large egg
- ½ sliced medium cucumber
- ¼ diced small red onion
- 1 tbsp olive oil
- 5 walnuts, halved
- Handful of watercress

INSTRUCTIONS:

1. Preheat oven to 400°F / 200°C. Wash and dry watercress.
2. Roast walnuts on a baking tray in the oven for 6 minutes.
3. Remove and cool.
4. Use sesame seeds, salt, and ghee to coat tuna.
5. Heat a griddle and fry as desired.
6. Remove and let cool for a bit before slicing.
7. Boil egg and place in cool water before peeling.
8. Slice the remaining ingredients.
9. Place everything atop the bed of watercress, and top with olive oil and mayo. Serve and enjoy.

Dinner - Steak Taco Bowl (See page 77)

DAY 18

Breakfast - Mango Smoothie (See page 49)
Lunch - Salmon and Vegetables (See page 53)
Dinner - Everything Bowl

Carbs: 4 grams
Protein: 32 grams
Fat: 43 grams
Calories: 558kcal

INGREDIENTS:

- ♦ 4.4 oz. / 125g lupin flakes
- ♦ 2 1/2 cup spinach, chopped
- ♦ 1 cup chicken broth
- ♦ 1 ½ sliced white mushrooms
- ♦ 1 tbsp ghee
- ♦ 1 drained can of pink salmon
- ♦ ¼ cup butter
- ♦ Sea salt
- ♦ 1 minced garlic clove
- ♦ 4 tbsp hulled hemp seeds
- ♦ 1 sliced large avo
- ♦ 2 tbsp olive oil

INSTRUCTIONS:

1. Start by cleaning and slicing mushrooms.
2. Place lupin flakes into bowl and pour broth over.
3. Stir and let sit for 15 minutes.
4. Remove spinach stems and finely chop, and mince garlic as well.
5. Heat half of the ghee over high heat in a frying pan, and saute garlic and spinach until soft.
6. Remove and cook mushrooms in the same pan.
7. Microwave lupin flakes for 2 mins after they have sit.
8. Place butter once done to melt, and fluff with fork before serving.
9. Slice avocado, and arrange all components into a bowl as desired. Serve and enjoy.

DAY 19

Breakfast - Caprese Omelet

Carbs: 4 grams
Protein: 30 grams
Fat: 44 grams
Calories: 533kcal

INGREDIENTS:

- 3 eggs
- ⅓ cup halved cherry tomatoes
- 1 tbsp butter
- 6 chopped basil leaves
- 2 fresh mozzarella slices
- 1 tbsp pesto
- 1 tbsp parmesan, grated
- Salt and pepper

INSTRUCTIONS:

1. Whisk eggs together with 1 tablespoon of water in a bowl.
2. Place a skillet on low heat and melt the butter.
3. Pour the eggs into the skillet and continually lift to make sure they don't stick.
4. When the eggs just become firm, place half of the tomatoes, the parmesan, basil, and mozzarella on one side.
5. Fold in half and cook until desired.
6. Top with pesto and the rest of the tomatoes, and serve.

Lunch - Chicken Salad (See page 76)
Dinner - Broccoli and Chicken Stir Fry (See page 60)

DAY 20

Breakfast - Hummus Breakfast Bowl (See page 48)
Lunch - Zucchini Pasta Alfredo

Carbs: 8 grams
Protein: 15 grams
Fat: 73 grams
Calories: 743kcal

INGREDIENTS:

- ♦ 2.65 pounds / 1.2kg spiralized zucchini
- ♦ 4 tbsp olive oil
- ♦ ¾ cup butter, unsalted
- ♦ 2 minced garlic cloves
- ♦ 6 oz. / 170g parmesan
- ♦ 6 oz. / 170g cream cheese
- ♦ 1 tsp oregano, chopped
- ♦ ¾ cups shredded cheddar
- ♦ 1 tbsp chopped basil
- ♦ Salt and pepper

INSTRUCTIONS:

1. Use a spiralizer to shred zucchini.
2. Place into a colander in the sink, sprinkle salt and let drain.
3. Melt butter in a pan, then add garlic and cook until soft.
4. Add cream and simmer.
5. And a handful of the shredded cheddar and the cream cheese, and stir until it all melts.
6. Keep adding the cheddar until all of it is melted.
7. Add the herbs and mix.
8. Remove sauce from heat and let thicken.
9. Pat the zucchini with a paper towel to dry.
10. Put olive oil in a frying pan and heat, and saute noodles.
11. Place the noodles in a large serving dish and mix with the alfredo sauce.
12. Top with parmesan and enjoy.

Dinner - Garlic & Honey Shrimp Fry (See page 62)

DAY 21

Breakfast - Vanilla Smoothie (See page 82)
Lunch - Burgers, Grass-Fed Style (See page 52)
Dinner - Crispy Thyme & Lemon Chicken

Carbs: 1 grams
Protein: 28 grams
Fat: 31 grams
Calories: 677kcal

INGREDIENTS:

- 8 boneless chicken thighs
- 2 tbsp lemon juice, fresh
- 1 tbsp chopped thyme
- 2 minced garlic cloves
- 1 tsp lemon zest
- 2 tbsp ghee
- 2 tbsp olive oil
- ¼ black pepper
- 1 tsp salt

INSTRUCTIONS:

1. Place thighs on a chopping board, skin side up, and flatten with a meat pounder.
2. Place them in a bowl and add lemon zest, juice, garlic, thyme, salt and pepper.
3. Coat evenly, and refrigerate for 1 hour minimum.
4. Place on a paper towel to dry.
5. Grease a large skillet with ghee and heat over medium-high.
6. Place thighs skin side down.
7. Cook for 10 minutes, then turn over and cook until done.
8. Place on a cooling rack and let rest before serving.

DAY 22

Breakfast - Full English Breakfast

Carbs: 7 grams
Protein: 30 grams
Fat: 55 grams
Calories: 658kcal

INGREDIENTS:

- 4 brown mushrooms
- 1 tbsp ghee
- 2 large eggs
- 5 thin bacon slices

- 4 cherry tomatoes
- ½ thawed frozen spinach
- Salt and pepper
- ½ sliced avocado

INSTRUCTIONS:

1. Use ghee to grease a skillet over medium heat.
2. Season mushrooms with salt and pepper while cooking bottom side up for 5 minutes.
3. Flip and cook for another 2 minutes, then move to a plate.
4. Fry the bacon as desired, then fry the eggs as desired.
5. Remove both, and fry the cherry tomatoes for about a minute.
6. Drain the spinach and cook in the same pan for a few seconds to soften.
7. Serve with the avocado and enjoy.

Lunch - Fish Tacos (See page 54)
Dinner - Italian Melt Omelet (See page 75)

DAY 23

Breakfast - Green Smoothie (See page 46)
Lunch - Tuna Salad

Carbs: 5 grams
Protein: 33 grams
Fat: 55 grams
Calories: 651kcal

INGREDIENTS:

- 1 tbsp lemon juice
- ¼ cup mayo
- 1 tbsp parsley, chopped
- 2 tbsp olive oil
- 1 romaine lettuce head
- Salt and pepper
- 1 medium cucumber
- ½ small red onion
- 1 drained jar of tuna
- 8 sliced olives
- 4 large eggs, hard-boiled

INSTRUCTIONS:

1. Place lemon juice, mayo, olive oil, salt, pepper, and parsley into a mason jar.
2. Close and shake until fully combined.
3. Slice the onion, cucumber, and olives, and place lettuce leaves into bowl.
4. Add onion, cucumber, olives, and tina.
5. Cut eggs into quarters and add to bowl.
6. Shake dressing again before drizzling onto salad. Serve and enjoy.

Dinner - Cod & Moroccan Couscous (See page 64)

DAY 24

Breakfast - French Toast (See page 50)
Lunch - Turkey Burrito Skillet (See page 56)
Dinner - Chicken and Blackberry Salad

Carbs: 7 grams
Protein: 48 grams
Fat: 40 grams
Calories: 600kcal

INGREDIENTS:

- 2 skinless chicken breasts
- 1 tsp thyme
- ¼ lemon, juiced
- 2 small lettuce heads
- ¼ cup olive oil
- ¼ cup black olives
- ½ cup canned artichoke hearts
- 1 blackberries, fresh
- 1 tbsp lemon juice
- Sea salt

INSTRUCTIONS:

1. Brush half of the olive oil over chicken, and add thyme and lemon juice.
2. Season with salt and let sit for 30 minutes.
3. Preheat oven to 400°F / 200°C.
4. Bake chicken in a baking dish for 30 minutes, and let cool when finished.
5. Wash lettuce and place into a serving bowl.
6. Sliced drained artichoke hearts and add them to the bowl with the chicken.
7. Add olives, and washed blackberries. Serve and enjoy.

DAY 25

Breakfast - Chocolate Smoothie

Carbs: 4 grams
Protein: 35 grams
Fat: 47 grams
Calories: 576kcal

INGREDIENTS:

- ¼ cup heavy whipping cream
- 2 large eggs
- 1 tbsp coconut oil
- ¼ cup plain or chocolate whey
- 5 drops stevia extract
- 1 tbsp cacao powder, unsweetened
- ¼ cup water
- Some ice cubes

INSTRUCTIONS:

1. Add all ingredients to a blender and blend until smooth and combined. Serve and enjoy.

Lunch - Bacon Wrapped Chicken Parcels (See page 86)
Dinner - Everything Bowl (See page 93)

DAY 26

Breakfast - Hummus Breakfast Bowl (See page 48)
Lunch - Mediterranean Chicken Risotto

Carbs: 6 grams
Protein: 42 grams
Fat: 33 grams
Calories: 513kcal

INGREDIENTS:

- ◆ 4 chicken breasts
- ◆ 1 small cauliflower head
- ◆ ½ cup pesto
- ◆ ¼ cup heavy whipping cream
- ◆ 1 ½ tsp lemon zest
- ◆ 2 crushed garlic cloves
- ◆ 2 tbsp ghee
- ◆ 2 tbsp basil, chopped
- ◆ Salt and pepper

INSTRUCTIONS:

1. Remove center and leaves from cauliflower to prepare for rice.
2. Cut into florets, wash, and drain proper.
3. Grate when dried, or pulse in a food processor.
4. Cut the chicken into bite-sized pieced.
5. Grease a pan with ghee, and place the chicken in it.
6. Cook for 15 minutes, then place aside.
7. Peel and mash garlic.
8. Use more ghee to grease another pan, and add lemon zest and garlic.
9. Cook over medium heat until brown.
10. Add cauliflower rice, and cook on high for 3 minutes.
11. Add parmesan and mix thoroughly. Serve and enjoy.

Dinner - Broccoli and Chicken Stir Fry (See page 60)

DAY 27

Breakfast - Green Smoothie (See page 46)
Lunch - Sardine Stuffed Avocado (See page 83)
Dinner - Bacon Hash & Wholegrain Mustard

Carbs: 5 grams
Protein: 20 grams
Fat: 47 grams
Calories: 522kcal

INGREDIENTS:

- 4 cups white mushrooms, sliced
- 12 bacon slices
- 1 tbsp orange zest
- 1 tbsp lemon juice
- 1 tbsp wholegrain mustard
- 1 tbsp ghee
- ¼ cup heavy whipping cream
- Salt and pepper

INSTRUCTIONS:

1. Chop the bacon and slice the mushrooms, then add bacon to a medium skillet greased with ghee.
2. Cook until slightly golden.
3. Add mushrooms and cook for 4 minutes.
4. Add orange zest and combine.
5. Add lemon juice, mustard, cream, and cook until sauce becomes thick.
6. Remove from heat, serve, and enjoy.

Breakfast - California Omelet

Carbs: 5 grams
Protein: 35 grams
Fat: 48 grams
Calories: 615kcal

INGREDIENTS:

- 6 eggs
- ¼ tsp sriracha
- ¼ tsp lemon juice
- 3 tbsp butter
- Salt and pepper
- 2 tbsp parsley, minced

- 10 deveined, peeled, cooked shrimp
- 1 sliced onion
- ¼ cup red bell pepper, minced
- 1 avocado
- 2 bacon slices

INSTRUCTIONS:

1. Whisk eggs, sriracha, lemon juice, and salt in a small bowl.
2. Place butter in a large pan on medium heat.
3. When it melts, add eggs.
4. Cook until slightly firm, lifting the bottom periodically to prevent sticking.
5. Place the remaining ingredients on top of one half of the omelet.
6. Fold over, and cook until finished. Serve and enjoy.

Lunch - Tuna Bowl (See page 91)

(See page 91)

Dinner - Chorizo, Chicken, and Avocado Salad (See page 88)

(See page 88)

Wrapping Up

Congratulations! You've made it to the end. We hope that your journey through this book was an informative one and that you now have the confidence and know-how you need to start your intermittent fasting journey. Be sure to visit the chapters in this book every now and then to refresh your memory, or build up hope again when you think you're slipping up.

Happy fasting!

Disclaimer

This book contains opinions and ideas of the author and is meant to teach the reader informative and helpful knowledge while due care should be taken by the user in the application of the information provided. The instructions and strategies are possibly not right for every reader and there is no guarantee that they work for everyone. Using this book and implementing the information/recipes therein contained is explicitly your own responsibility and risk. This work with all its contents, does not guarantee correctness, completion, quality or correctness of the provided information. Misinformation or misprints cannot be completely eliminated.

Made in the USA
Las Vegas, NV
07 September 2021

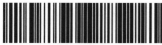